I0416077

What I need to know about Hepatitis B

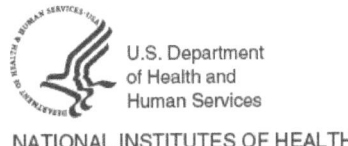

U.S. Department
of Health and
Human Services

NATIONAL INSTITUTES OF HEALTH

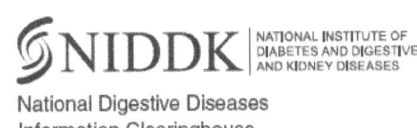

National Digestive Diseases
Information Clearinghouse

Contents

What is hepatitis B?

Hepatitis* B is a **virus,** or infection, that causes liver disease and **inflammation** of the liver. Viruses can cause sickness. For example, the flu is caused by a virus. People can pass viruses to each other.

Inflammation is swelling that occurs when tissues of the body become injured or infected. Inflammation can cause organs to not work properly.

What is the liver?

The liver is an organ that does many important things. You cannot live without a liver.

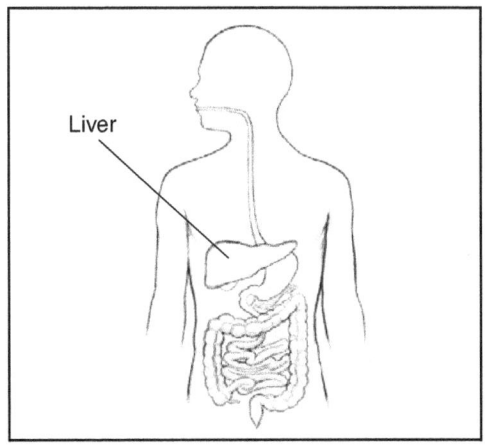

Hepatitis B is a virus, or infection, that causes liver disease and inflammation of the liver.

*See page 20 for tips on how to say the words in **bold** type.

1

The liver

- removes harmful chemicals from your blood
- fights infection
- helps digest food
- stores nutrients and vitamins
- stores energy

Who gets hepatitis B?

Anyone can get hepatitis B, but those more likely to are people who

- were born to a mother with hepatitis B
- are in contact with blood, needles, or body fluids at work
- live with someone who currently has an active hepatitis B infection
- have had more than one sex partner in the last 6 months or have a history of sexually transmitted disease

- are on kidney dialysis—the process of filtering wastes and extra water from the body by means other than the kidneys

- are taking medicines that suppress the immune system, such as steroids or chemotherapy medicines

- have lived in or travel often to parts of the world where hepatitis B is common

- are from Asian and Pacific Island nations

- are infected with HIV or hepatitis C

- have injected illegal drugs

- work or live in a prison

- had a blood transfusion or organ transplant before the mid-1980s

Also, men who have sex with men are more likely to get hepatitis B.

How could I get hepatitis B?

You could get hepatitis B through contact with an infected person's blood, semen, or other body fluid. This contact could occur by

- being born to a mother with hepatitis B

- getting an accidental stick with a needle that was used on an infected person

- having unprotected sex with an infected person

- having contact with blood or open sores of an infected person

- sharing drug needles or other drug materials with an infected person

- being tattooed or pierced with unsterilized tools that were used on an infected person

- using an infected person's razor, toothbrush, or nail clippers

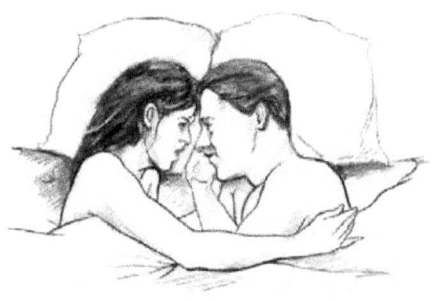

You could get hepatitis B from having unprotected sex with an infected person.

You cannot get hepatitis B from

- shaking hands or holding hands with an infected person

- being coughed or sneezed on by an infected person

- hugging an infected person

- sitting next to an infected person

- sharing spoons, forks, and other eating utensils

- drinking water or eating food

A baby cannot get hepatitis B from breast milk.

What are the symptoms of hepatitis B?

Most people do not have any symptoms of hepatitis B. Adults and children ages 5 and older may have one or more of the following symptoms:

- feeling tired
- muscle soreness
- upset stomach
- stomach pain
- fever
- loss of appetite
- diarrhea
- dark-yellow urine
- light-colored stools
- yellowish eyes and skin, called **jaundice**

When symptoms occur, they can begin 2 to 5 months after coming into contact with the virus. See a doctor right away if you or a child in your care has symptoms of hepatitis B.

What is acute hepatitis B?

Acute hepatitis B is a short-term infection with the hepatitis B virus. Symptoms usually last several weeks but they can last up to 6 months. The infection sometimes clears up because your body is able to fight off the infection and get rid of the virus. Most healthy adults and children older than 5 who have hepatitis B get better without treatment.

What is chronic hepatitis B?

Chronic hepatitis B is a long-lasting infection with the hepatitis B virus. Chronic hepatitis B occurs when the body can't get rid of the hepatitis B virus. Children, especially infants, are more likely to get chronic hepatitis B, which usually has no symptoms until signs of liver damage appear.

Without treatment, chronic hepatitis B can cause liver cancer or severe liver damage that leads to liver failure. Liver failure occurs when the liver stops working properly.

How is hepatitis B diagnosed?

A blood test will show if you have hepatitis B. Blood tests are done at a doctor's office or outpatient facility. A blood sample is taken using a needle inserted into a vein in your arm or hand. The blood sample is sent to a lab to test for hepatitis B.

If you are at higher risk of getting hepatitis B, get tested. If you are pregnant, you should also get tested. Many people with hepatitis B do not know they are infected. Early diagnosis and treatment can help prevent liver damage.

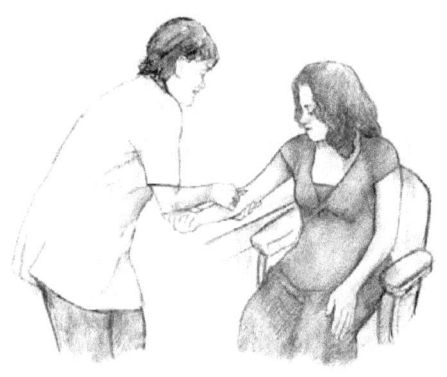

A blood test will show if you have hepatitis B.

Your doctor may suggest getting a liver **biopsy** if chronic hepatitis B is suspected. A liver biopsy is a test to take a small piece of your liver to look for liver damage. The doctor may ask you to stop taking certain medicines before the test. You may be asked to fast for 8 hours before the test.

During the test, you lie on a table with your right hand resting above your head. Medicine is applied to numb the area where the biopsy needle will be inserted. If needed, sedatives and pain medicine are also given. The doctor uses a needle to take a small piece of liver tissue. After the test, you must lie on your right side for up to 2 hours. You will stay 2 to 4 hours after the test before being sent home.

A liver biopsy is performed at a hospital or outpatient center by a doctor. The liver tissue is sent to a special lab where a doctor looks at the tissue with a microscope and sends a report to your doctor.

How is hepatitis B treated?

Hepatitis B is not usually treated unless it becomes chronic. Chronic hepatitis B is treated with medicines that slow or stop the virus from damaging the liver.

Medicines for Chronic Hepatitis B

Your doctor will choose medicines or a combination of medicines that are likely to work for you. The doctor will closely watch your symptoms and schedule regular blood tests to make sure treatment is working.

Medicines given by shots include

- **interferon**
- **peginterferon**

Medicines taken by mouth include

- **adefovir**
- **entecavir**
- **lamivudine**
- **telbivudine**
- **tenofovir**

The length of treatment varies. Talk with your doctor before taking other prescription medicines and over-the-counter medicines.

Liver Transplant

A liver transplant may be necessary if chronic hepatitis B causes severe liver damage that leads to liver failure. Symptoms of severe liver damage include the symptoms of hepatitis B and

- generalized itching

- a longer than usual amount of time for bleeding to stop

- easy bruising

- swollen stomach or ankles

- spiderlike blood vessels, called spider **angiomas,** that develop on the skin

Liver transplant is surgery to remove a diseased or injured liver and replace it with a healthy one from another person, called a donor. If your doctors tell you that you need a transplant, you should talk with them about the long-term demands of living with a liver transplant.

A team of surgeons—doctors who specialize in surgery—performs a liver transplant in a hospital. You will learn how to take care of yourself after you go home and about the medicines you'll need to take to protect your new liver. Medicines taken after liver transplant surgery can prevent hepatitis B from coming back.

Testing for Liver Cancer

Having hepatitis B increases your risk for getting liver cancer, so your doctor may suggest an ultrasound test of the liver every 6 to12 months. Finding cancer early makes it more treatable. Ultrasound is a machine that uses sound waves to create a picture of your liver. Ultrasound is performed at a hospital or radiology center by a specially trained technician. The image, called a sonogram, can show the liver's size and the presence of cancerous tumors.

How can I avoid getting hepatitis B?

You can avoid getting hepatitis B by receiving the hepatitis B **vaccine.**

Vaccines are medicines that keep you from getting sick. Vaccines teach the body to attack specific viruses and infections. The hepatitis B vaccine teaches your body to attack the hepatitis B virus.

Since the 1980s, a hepatitis B vaccine has been available and should be given to newborns and children in the United States. Adults at higher risk of getting hepatitis B should also get the vaccine.

The hepatitis B vaccine is given in three shots over 6 months. You must get all three hepatitis B vaccine shots to be fully protected.

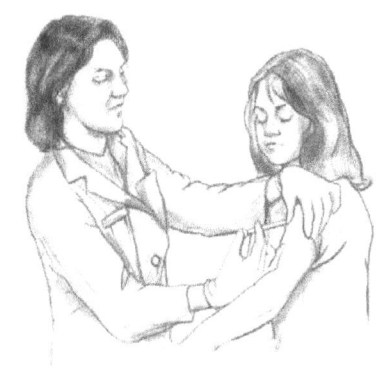

You can avoid getting hepatitis B
by receiving the hepatitis B vaccine.

If you are traveling to countries where hepatitis B is common, try to get all the shots before you go. If you don't have time to get all the shots before you travel, get as many as you can. Even one shot may provide some protection against the virus.

You can protect yourself and others from getting hepatitis B if you

- use a condom during sex
- do not share drug needles and other drug materials
- do not donate blood or blood products
- wear gloves if you have to touch another person's blood or open sores
- do not share or borrow a toothbrush, razor, or nail clippers
- make sure any tattoos or body piercings you get are done with sterile tools

- tell your doctor and your dentist if you have hepatitis B

If you are pregnant and have hepatitis B, tell the doctor and staff who deliver your baby. The hepatitis B vaccine and hepatitis B immune globulin should be given to your baby right after birth. The vaccine will greatly reduce the chance of your baby getting the infection.

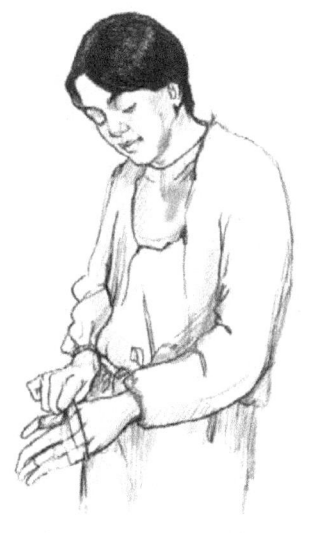

Wear gloves if you have to touch another person's blood or open sores.

What should I do if I think I have been in contact with the hepatitis B virus?

See your doctor right away if you think you have been in contact with the hepatitis B virus. A dose of the hepatitis B vaccine taken with a medicine called hepatitis B immune globulin may protect you from getting sick if taken shortly after coming into contact with the hepatitis B virus.

Eating, Diet, and Nutrition

If you have chronic hepatitis B, you should do things to take care of yourself, including eating a healthy diet. Avoid drinking alcohol, which can harm the liver. Talk with your doctor before taking vitamins and other supplements.

Points to Remember

- Hepatitis B is a virus, or infection, that causes liver disease and inflammation of the liver.

- Anyone can get hepatitis B, but some people are more likely to than others.

- You could get hepatitis B through contact with an infected person's blood, semen, or other body fluid.

- Most people do not have any symptoms of hepatitis B. Adults and children ages 5 and older may have symptoms.

- See a doctor right away if you or a child in your care has symptoms of hepatitis B.

- Acute hepatitis B is a short-term infection with the hepatitis B virus.

- Chronic hepatitis B is a long-lasting infection with the hepatitis B virus. Chronic hepatitis B occurs when the body can't get rid of the hepatitis B virus.

- Children, especially infants, are more likely to get chronic hepatitis B.

- A blood test will show if you have hepatitis B.

- If you are at higher risk of getting hepatitis B, get tested. If you are pregnant, you should also get tested.

- Many people with hepatitis B do not know they are infected. Early diagnosis and treatment can help prevent liver damage.

- Hepatitis B is usually not treated unless it becomes chronic. Chronic hepatitis B is treated with medicines that slow or stop the virus from damaging the liver.

- You can avoid getting hepatitis B by receiving the hepatitis B vaccine.

- Tell your doctor and your dentist if you have hepatitis B.

- If you are pregnant and have hepatitis B, tell the doctor and staff who deliver your baby.

- See your doctor right away if you think you have been in contact with the hepatitis B virus.

Hope through Research

The National Institute of Diabetes and Digestive and Kidney Diseases (NIDDK) conducts and supports basic and clinical research into many digestive disorders, including hepatitis B. A team of NIDDK researchers is studying individuals who have been diagnosed with hepatitis B to identify factors that affect how the disease progresses. To improve current knowledge about the disease and long-term outcomes, the Hepatitis B Research Network is collecting health and disease information from these individuals. The study is funded under NIH clinical trial number NCT01306071.

Participants in clinical trials can play a more active role in their own health care, gain access to new research treatments before they are widely available, and help others by contributing to medical research. For information about current studies, visit *www.ClinicalTrials.gov.*

Pronunciation Guide

adefovir (ad-DEF-oh-vihr)

angiomas (an-jee-OH-muhs)

biopsy (BY-op-see)

chronic (KRON-ik)

entecavir (INT-ih-CAH-vihr)

hepatitis (HEP-uh-TY-tiss)

inflammation (IN-fluh-MAY-shuhn)

interferon (IN-tur-FIHR-on)

jaundice (JAWN-diss)

lamivudine (luh-MIH-vyoo-deen)

peginterferon (PEG-IN-tur-FIHR-on)

telbivudine (tel-BIH-vyoo-deen)

tenofovir (te-NOH-foh-vihr)

vaccine (vak-SEEN)

virus (VY-ruhss)

For More Information

American Liver Foundation
39 Broadway, Suite 2700
New York, NY 10006
Phone: 1–800–GO–Liver (1–800–465–4837)
    or 212–668–1000
Fax: 212–483–8179
Email: info@liverfoundation.org
Internet: www.liverfoundation.org

Hepatitis B Foundation
3805 Old Easton Road
Doylestown, PA 18902
Phone: 215–489–4900
Fax: 215–489–4920
Email: contact@hepb.org
Internet: www.hepb.org

Hepatitis Foundation International
504 Blick Drive
Silver Spring, MD 20904
Phone: 1–800–891–0707 or 301–622–4200
Fax: 301–622–4702
Email: info@hepatitisfoundation.org
Internet: www.hepfi.org

National Center for HIV/AIDS, Viral Hepatitis, STD, and TB Prevention
Centers for Disease Control and Prevention
1600 Clifton Road
Atlanta, GA 30333
Phone: 1–800–CDC–INFO (1–800–232–4636)
TTY: 1–888–232–6348
Email: cdcinfo@cdc.gov
Internet: www.cdc.gov/nchhstp

The National Digestive Diseases Information Clearinghouse (NDDIC) also has booklets about hepatitis A, hepatitis C, and liver transplantation:

- *What I need to know about Hepatitis A*

- *What I need to know about Hepatitis C*

- *What I need to know about Liver Transplantation*

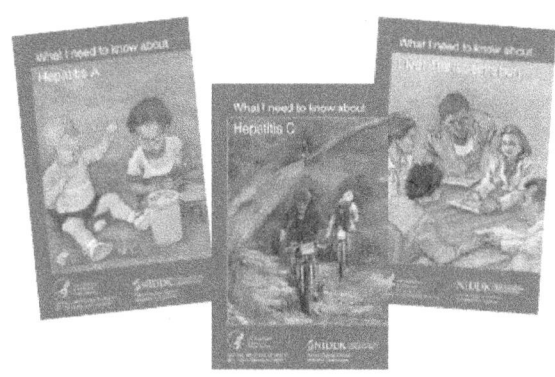

You can get a free copy of each booklet by calling 1–800–891–5389, by going online to *www.catalog.niddk.nih.gov,* or by writing to

NDDIC
2 Information Way
Bethesda, MD 20892–3570

Hepatitis information for health professionals is also available.

Acknowledgments

Publications produced by the Clearinghouse are carefully reviewed by both NIDDK scientists and outside experts. The NDDIC would like to thank the following individuals for providing scientific and editorial review or facilitating field-testing of the original version of this publication:

Bruce Bacon, M.D.
American Liver Foundation
New York, NY

Theo Heller, M.D.
NIDDK, National Institutes of Health
Bethesda, MD

Luby Garza-Abijaoude, M.S., R.D., L.D.
Texas Department of Health
Austin, TX

Thelma Thiel, R.N.
Hepatitis Foundation International
Cedar Grove, NJ

National Digestive Diseases Information Clearinghouse

2 Information Way
Bethesda, MD 20892–3570
Phone: 1–800–891–5389
TTY: 1–866–569–1162
Fax: 703–738–4929
Email: nddic@info.niddk.nih.gov
Internet: www.digestive.niddk.nih.gov

The National Digestive Diseases Information Clearinghouse (NDDIC) is a service of the National Institute of Diabetes and Digestive and Kidney Diseases (NIDDK). The NIDDK is part of the National Institutes of Health of the U.S. Department of Health and Human Services. Established in 1980, the Clearinghouse provides information about digestive diseases to people with digestive disorders and to their families, health care professionals, and the public. The NDDIC answers inquiries, develops and distributes publications, and works closely with professional and patient organizations and Government agencies to coordinate resources about digestive diseases.

This publication may contain information about medications. When prepared, this publication included the most current information available. For updates or for questions about any medications, contact the U.S. Food and Drug Administration toll-free at 1–888–INFO–FDA (1–888–463–6332) or visit *www.fda.gov.* Consult your health care provider for more information.

www.ingramcontent.com/pod-product-compliance
Lightning Source LLC
Chambersburg PA
CBHW070940290526
45795CB00003B/1098